GET IN SHAPE

SMALL STEPS FOR BIG RESULTS

SIMPLE AND EFFECTIVE GUIDE TO HELP YOU LOSE WEIGHT, FEEL ENERGIZED, GET IN SHAPE AND STAY IN SHAPE

Copyright © 2020

All right is reserved. No part of this book may be reproduced or used in any manner without written permission of the copyright owner except for the use of quotations in a book review.

You can also follow me here on Facebook

https://www.facebook.com/RichardRobertson40/

To stay updated with our latest news and new book releases.

Table of Contents

Introduction 1

Chapter 1 : The Fundamentals of Getting in Shape 5

    Motivation and Mindset 6

    The "fixed" Mindset 7

    The "growth" Mindset 8

    Sticking to Good Habits.. 11

Chapter 2 : Eating Right to Get in Shape 13

    Best Foods to Get in Shape 19

Chapter 3 : Setting Up A Get in Shape Exercise Program 23

Chapter 4 : Importance of Rest and Sleep 27

Chapter 5 : Stress Free Weight Loss 31

Chapter 6 : Exercises to Help you Get in Shape 33

    Weighted T-Exercise 33

    Sit-ups 34

    Dumbbell Press 35

    Hamstrings/Back 36

    Stability Hip Raise 37

    Speed Walk 38

Dumbbell flyes 39

Triceps Press 40

Seated Arm Stretch 42

Kettlebell/Dumbbell Goblet Squat 43

Leg Raise 44

One Arm Rowing 45

American Swing 46

Dumbbell Pushup Pulls 47

Leg Raise Bridge 49

Abdominal Plank 51

Lunge Reach Stretch 52

Single Leg Calf Raise 53

Mountain Runners 55

Glute Lift 55

Bicycle crunches 56

Side Crunch 58

Side Plank 59

Plank Ups 60

Jump squats 62

Chapter 7 : Tips to Get Motivated 64

Journals and calendars are your friends 64

Get rid of negativity 64

Surround yourself with motivation 65

Have a goal in mind 65

Group activities aren't always bad 66

Schedules 66

Tell yourself that working out is fun! 67

Don't fight the addiction 67

Playlists and audiobooks 68

Everything's a competition 68

Television 68

Start small 69

Remember why you are doing it 69

Motivate others 69

Post-workout analysis 70

Chapter 8 : Measure Your Progress 71
   Take Periodic Photos 72

Measure Your Body Parts 73

What If the Results Are Not Productive? 74

Chapter 9 : Achieving Amazing Results 77
   Work at it Each Day 77

Don't Quit 78

Don't Allow Failure to Win 78

It's in the Mind 78

Change It Up 79
Don't Forget a Rest Day 80
The power of "a plan" 80
The Power of Persistence 81
Positive Energy 81
Take Action 83
High Achievement 83
Discipline 84

Chapter 10 : How to Stay in Shape Forever 87
Eating Right + Exercise = Good Shape 87

Conclusion 93

INTRODUCTION

Weight is something we all struggle with, but it doesn't have to be this way. Getting in shape is easier than it seems, although it does require a commitment from you. This book will show you how you can get in shape because it uses practical advice. We are often confused about how exactly to get in shape but once you know how to do this, it's a lot easier.

Many people start off great with their exercises and eating plan but then quickly fall off of it. This is a common problem because we live in a society that expects instant results. It takes time to lose weight and get in shape; however, you can begin this process in as little as seven days. You have to be ready to commit to weight loss and do what it takes to reduce your weight. The weight isn't going to come off on its own; you have to do some work. If you go into it thinking that there's some magic bullet, you're going to be disappointed in your results.

Get in shape Small steps for big results

Excessive weight can definitely be an obstacle in life daily. This is simply the harsh reality. Although you don't want to give people the time of day who treat you differently, it's a weird world out there and sometimes it's just easier to not have an extra thing that people can judge you on, sigh.

You could feel held back in your job or excluded in a social environment, and ideally you really don't want to or need to be slowed down in life while carrying that extra load. That load I'm talking about is physical and mental — that's double the stress.

For many, making changes to a lifestyle you have been comfortable with for so long can be extremely difficult. It means looking at the lifestyle which you live and being brutally honest with yourself and those supporting you, regarding the habits you have now and the ones you want to change.

However, the truth of the matter is that you don't necessarily have to make many dramatic changes all at once to get in shape. It is far easier and better to change one habit at a time. Once you have incorporated one easy habit into your lifestyle, it becomes an essential part of your routine, and it makes it easier to incorporate a new healthy habit. This way, it becomes easier for you to lose weight, get in shape, and feel better about yourself.

Losing weight is not just about being accepted, though it can be the obstacle that you beat that proves you can overcome anything in life and achieve many other goals.

Add to this the obvious health benefits. People that take care of themselves will live a lot longer, be a lot more active, full of life, and get a lot more done in their lifetime. In other words, take care of your body and it will take care of you by making you feel great!

You also have to be ready for at least some moderate activity. You need to move to keep your metabolism high which makes it easier to burn calories and keep the weight from coming back. If you're not going to be active, it will be tougher to see any sustained weight loss because your body simply needs movement for you to be successful.

You can lose weight on your own, but at times it gets hard. That's when it's good to look for a support system to help you out. A good support system is essential – the stronger it is, the easier it will be to accomplish your goals. Your family and your friends, and anyone who is undertaking the same journey as you, will certainly play an essential role in your success.

Get in shape Small steps for big results

There's a lot that goes on with you emotionally when you try to lose weight. If you don't have anyone there to back you up, your chances of failure are that much greater. A good support system can make a world of difference. With a great support system, you'll have the incentive you need to lose weight and you'll get that motivation which will help you stick with it.

Having goals will give you something to strive for. It might be to lose 15 pounds in a couple of months or be able to run several miles or even a marathon. Whatever you want to do, you need to write it down and make goals a part of your daily routine to help you stay on track.

There are two factors for losing weight and keeping it off–eating right and weight-loss exercise–which this book will give you some easy tips to follow.

Getting in shape doesn't have to be a complex thing it can be done by anyone. All you need is to be ready for the process and to commit yourself to it. Use this guide to get in shape and feel better than you have in a long time.

CHAPTER 1

THE FUNDAMENTALS OF GETTING IN SHAPE

The truth is, almost any diet and exercise plan when followed consistently will get you into better shape. The crucial ingredient to getting there is forming the right habits, learning to maintain those habits, and breaking the bad habits that are holding you back.

You have heard people who live very healthy lives say, "It's not a diet; it's a lifestyle." These are people who have ingrained healthy habits into their way of living. They no longer have to work so hard to be healthy, now it's just who they are. The truth is, that once you change your habits, and healthy habits are your new normal, your current bad habits will sound awful to you.

So, the way to get in shape is not through choosing the right magic supplement, or the right fad diet. The way to get into shape is to become a new person. A new person who moves more every day than you do now, a person who eats fewer calories than you currently do, and a person who gets those calories from real, unprocessed, whole foods. BOOM!!!

Motivation and Mindset

If getting in great shape was easy, everyone would have a perfect body. It is not easy, but it is one of those rare things that if you do the work, you can literally see and feel the payoff 24/7/365.

As you begin physical training it is critical to understand the powerful role your mindset plays in whether you succeed or fail. You are attempting to make a big change in your life, and thinking the wrong way about this decision can really affect how far you go.

One of my most important tasks in this first chapter is to help you understand how your mindset can either be a big asset in your quest for fitness, or the thing that makes you part of the 90% who quit.

On the other hand, there are people who mobilize the power of their mind to generate success in new and complex undertakings. This is where you want to be.

The "fixed" Mindset

Why do people avoid doing something they know will be good for them?

One of the things that I believe stops many people in their tracks is not believing they can do something. Each of us has ideas in our mind that create our personal reality. These are things we believe but are not necessarily true. These ideas can cause us a lot of problems.

First are the expectations that people have when they begin a program. Many people will begin a fitness program unconsciously expecting to fail!

These ideas, and variations of them, conspire to limit the chances of someone's success before they even start to work.

This is called a fixed mindset. It means that people believe they can determine in advance how successful they will be at any endeavor.

The common theme in all these ideas is that the person thinks they know in advance how successful they will be at something before they even try to do it!

People with fixed mindsets accept huge limitations on their potential before they make an attempt.

The "growth" Mindset

This means that you will only find out how successful you can be by working persistently at something.

People who have a growth mindset take on a new task believing "It will be difficult, but I can do this." When you have a growth mindset you approach the task knowing it may be difficult, but you are committed to giving it your best shot.

For now, in terms of your physical fitness, realize that there is no way to tell in advance how strong, agile, resilient, and capable you can become. That is to be determined by your hard work and persistence. How far you can go will only be discovered through unrelenting work.

If you have lost control or simply fancied something that you couldn't resist, just accept it and move on. Remember, you're in control. Many people eat more because they are unhappy, so while they aren't getting any closer to their goals and are still overweight it can cause them to be upset further and to keep eating, which is a never-ending cycle of emotions that gets you nowhere.

If this is what you're like, and you're feeling depressed, then try to flip your emotions. Instead of being unhappy, think about how happy you will be when you have reached your goal and be happy right now in belief that you will get there for real.

As you know, you will not lose weight overnight so it's good to keep the mindset that every day counts even if you can't see it on the scale. Just think of it as one big step closer–even if it feels like a small step. I would advise you to not weigh yourself every day as this may throw you off and any progress may seem like it's happening too slowly. Stick to once a week at the same time in the morning. If you do weigh yourself at different times, do not be alarmed if you seem to have put on weight as it can and will fluctuate during the day and throughout the week. This is because of things you consume and how your body handles them.

What you can also do is look at it as a game or challenge so that it becomes enjoyable rather than something you hate. The best way to do this is to find another person or a group to share your progress with. This can be friends or family or even people you don't know, and sometimes a group. Because you have the same goals as other people out there and it's also a great way to make some new friends.

You can make certain meals feel like a treat even though they are nowhere near as bad as some of your usual eating habits, but they can still fill that desire. Moderation and better choices come into play here so don't go out and order that burger and fries. Have a chicken salad instead.

Every time you look in the fridge and spot something that you really shouldn't be eating, think of that food in the future and not the present. In the present it may taste nice but soon after in the future you will feel guilty and a few days after that the scales may not show the progress you wanted it to show, so just think ahead in time before making any decisions when making food choices.

People may make fun of you for choosing to diet and exercise, and they may not believe in you for whatever reason. This may be because they could not imagine themselves changing their lifestyle in such a way so in their eyes you must also fail at it. Shrug it off and continue as normal, and you will be the one laughing when you reach your goals. It's not an issue of what other people think as it's your own actions that dictates your outcome. To achieve this, you need to let go of all your fears that could make it more difficult for you and just concentrate on the end result.

Sometimes when you are doing well you may treat yourself a little too much and then it backfires, and you end up doing more damage to your progress than you would have imagined. Instead of treating yourself to something bad to eat, you could challenge yourself to have something healthy in place of the treat and then feel twice as good later. Self-satisfaction is the biggest reward. Remember, it's still completely fine to treat yourself now and then to avoid binging. Have a cheat meal or a cheat day but fit it into your daily calorie limit.

Sticking to Good Habits

Most people want to be the best person they can be. They want to live healthy, well-rounded lives that satisfy them. In fact, they usually all know what they SHOULD be doing on a day-to-day basis to achieve the life they desire. So why is it so difficult to stick to good habits? Why do we get motivated in the beginning only to fall back into bad habits a short time later?

Have you ever resolved to add a healthy habit to your life? Lose 20 pounds? Eat healthier? Increase the amount of weight you can lift? Chances are if you are like most, you started those practices with the best intentions, only to get sidetracked somewhere along the way and they never became habits. Why does that happen so consistently to so many of us? The answer is that we try to make changes the wrong way. By trying to make a change in the wrong way, there is little possibility of it ever becoming a lasting change or habit. This book will show you a better strategy to finally successfully make long-term changes in your life.

CHAPTER 2

EATING RIGHT TO GET IN SHAPE

Getting in shape starts with looking at your food and how much you are eating. One of the many reasons why some people find they can't lose weight is because they have difficulty when it comes to how much they should be consuming.

Feeling like you are on a diet can make some people anxious and stressed, and measuring can be even more restrictive. However, there is a simple way to ensure that you are allocating the right amount of food to your plate. Simply fill one half of your plate with your vegetables and then divide the other half into two equal portions for your carbohydrates and protein servings.

Eating right starts with cooking right. Healthy food preparation must begin at home. Learn to cook tasty, low-calorie meals which are most of all, easy to prepare.

If food doesn't look appetizing on your plate or table, it will not be eaten. Food should be a whole experience satisfying all the senses. Food presentation is very important. Make food look opulent by using the fine china or silverware. Dress up the table with a colorful tablecloth, fresh flowers, and candles.

This simple way ensures that you don't have to stress out on measuring weights and also ensures that you get the right serving sizes.

When it comes to vegetables, many people become bored eating the same thing over and over. Carrots may taste great for the first few nights, but after a week it can get boring and you may find yourself reaching for something less healthy. Not only that, but you can also lose out on the essential nutrients found in other vegetables that your body needs. Instead, stop dishing up the same old vegetables and try a wide range of items.

Vary the way you cook your vegetables; some can be eaten raw, some boiled, some steamed, some grilled, or even baked. Make sure they have been cooked to an al dente state. When you overcook your vegetables, they lose their nutritional values and so your body won't get the essential vitamins and minerals it needs to stay healthy.

Get in shape Small steps for big results

The best way to cook vegetables as you are undergoing your weight loss journey is to steam or sauté them. Avoid microwaving them as they lose their vitamin contents and reduce their flavor, as well as the steaming in the bag method.

Preparing food can be fun though and will open your taste buds to new flavors that aren't as bad for you as what you may consume from takeaways and fast food restaurants. I'm going to go through some foods that you should be eating as well as how to deal with choosing beverages.

Eat fresh, unprocessed foods; anything that comes in a tin or sold as a microwave meal or TV dinner is most likely not good for you at all. Most of the time they have high sugar and salt content which you don't want to consume in excessive amounts. Salt makes you retain water making you feel fatter and sugar increases insulin levels making you hungry again.

If you want to jump straight in and be strict from the start, then stick to a clean diet full of fresh food. This may require that you go shopping more often as fresh food doesn't last as long as frozen or tinned foods, but that can be a good thing so that you won't have extra food in the cabinet waiting on you to give in to some heavy midnight snacking. You can buy what you need for the day, or even a couple of days, and then there's less chance of overeating.

Empty your cabinet of everything bad for you and proceed to throw it away or give it away. If you want to be more selective in terms of what treats you give up, make a list of snacks and cut out any that contain an insane amount of calories compared to others. Rather than cutting out everything, if it's one of your daily choices it will still make a noticeable impact.

A lot of people drink their extra calories on and don't even realize it. This can be through fizzy drinks, fruit juice, or even milk. I would advise you to make the switch to drinking ice cold water. It may seem like a joke to some people and they may even laugh at the idea, but you can have the last laugh because water has no calories and can actually help you burn fat. It's extremely healthy and just what your body needs. Just make sure you drink 6-8 glasses a day and you will feel better for it. And, it's actually refreshing as well. Once you get used to it, you're not likely to go back. I wouldn't cut out milk completely but cut back to skimmed milk or 1% fat milk, depending on your preference for your cereals and hot drinks.

Another hot drink I would recommend is green tea, which much like ice cold water is known to raise your metabolism and contains no calories. There's a whole range of other flavors of tea you could try out to satisfy your taste buds if you're getting bored of the green variety, and these still make for a much better choice than fizzy soda or fruit drinks. Peppermint and chamomile really allow me to relax and can be something to sip when you may have picked up a snack.

Alcohol has a lot of calories in it and is often full of sugar. It also slows down the rate at which you burn calories, so if you really want to lose weight you should cut it out completely. You will feel a lot better for it, but if you must drink to keep your sanity, I would say drink in moderation and make up for it with extra exercise. It's best to stay away from it though, as I know for sure once you start it's hard to stop and then, because it lowers your blood sugar levels, it makes you hungry and makes it more difficult to resist bad snacks afterwards.

Fat and carbs are often made out to be the enemy, but the truth is that not all of them are bad. A balanced diet is perfect for keeping you full, satisfied, and never too bored while trying to lose weight.

When looking at what carbs you should eat, remember that the simple carbs like white rice, white bread, and white potatoes should be avoided if possible. Snacks can also contain a lot of simple carbs.

Fruits are best consumed whole and not as a juice because the whole fruit will give you all the fiber. The fiber found in complex carbs is beneficial to you as it keeps you fuller longer in comparison to a food containing simple carbs, so that means less hunger pains and no overeating.

For breakfast, it's good to have a healthy cereal — but be warned as some cereals have a lot of sugar added to them. You want to choose one that is more on the pure and natural side.

If you usually have fried eggs, have them poached or boiled instead. If you must have bacon, then do it on the grill and try bacon medallions instead as they have all the fat trimmed off.

Snacks are not as bad as you may think. In fact, they can actually be a good way to keep you going until the next meal — especially if you have been exercising and need a bit of energy, but trying to stick to the healthy stuff such as fruit. If you're looking to try something a little different, but still good for you. Ryvita crackers and rice cakes are good alternatives to potato chips. Cottage cheese or quark cheese is perfect for these types of snacks also and is a lot healthier than regular cheese, which I try to cut down on when watching my calorie intake.

If you have to eat savory snacks and chocolates while you get used to dieting or if you simply can't give them up, then check out the weight watchers range. Calories, fat, and sugar are usually reduced quite a lot, which helps if you're used to eating the alternative higher calorie brands.

Best Foods to Get in Shape

Oats. Oats will give you energy and strength. Oats contain insoluble fiber that boosts your metabolism and makes you feel full longer.

Green Tea. Green tea contains catechins that increase your metabolism and help you burn more fat.

Almonds and other nuts. Almond contains dietary fiber who contributes to the sensation of being full. Almonds and nuts are good fat and increase energy and metabolism.

Bananas. Bananas contain pectin which keeps you feeling fuller longer. Bananas are full of essential nutrients that you need to stay healthy.

Apples. Like bananas, apples contain pectin that makes you feel full longer. They also contain flavonoids that burn fat and are full of vitamin C, dietary fiber, and antioxidants.

Broccoli. Broccoli is full of fiber and vitamins. Broccoli also contains sulforaphane which causes fat loss. It's one of the healthiest vegetables.

Salmon. Salmon is full of omega 3, and omega-3 fatty acids reduce fat. Salmon also contains lots of protein. High-protein foods are natural fat burners.

Berries. Berries are strong antioxidants and contain pectin like apples and bananas that keeps you feeling fuller longer.

Eggs. Eggs contain lots of vitamins and minerals. They also contain calcium and are a good source of protein.

More healthy foods. Almond milk, apricot, asparagus, avocado, beans and lentils, brown rice, brussels sprouts, cabbage, carrots, cauliflower, cherries, chia seeds, chicken breast, coconut, coffee, dark chocolate, flaxseed, garlic, grapes, kale, kiwi, lean beef, lemons, mangoes, olive oil, onions, oranges, papaya, peaches, peanut butter, pineapple, popcorn, pumpkin, quinoa, sardines, spinach, sweet potatoes, tomatoes, and tuna.

Get in shape Small steps for big results

By learning to eat sensibly and developing ways to stay motivated while changing some lifestyle habits, and exercising, you'll find that weight loss can be achieved fast. These things may sound like lofty ideals prescribed by every fitness expert and health guru. Probably – yes; however, with knowledge of nutrition comes understanding. Strive to be wise consumers, informed cooks, nutrition experts, and fitness seekers. Don't throw out everything in the kitchen and start from scratch. That is unrealistic. Simply learn the principles of eating complete meals every 3-4 hours and learn to balance protein, fats, and carbohydrates at those meals.

When most people go on a diet, the first thing they do is eliminate the carbohydrates. Like potatoes and bread, and that's when pasta becomes the enemy. But actually, in moderation these foods provide energy and when balanced with protein they can lead to weight loss.

Here is the breakdown of a complete meal:

- ❖ 60% CARBOHYDRATES – this includes fruits, vegetables, and whole grains–mainly everything in the produce section or foods that are in their whole state.
- ❖ 20% PROTEIN – needed to develop and maintain muscle tone.

- ❖ 20% FAT – each meal needs to include good fats like olive oil, macadamia nut oil, nuts, and seeds like ground flaxseeds. Fat is necessary to keep our hair shiny and our skin youthful looking and our joints lubricated plus it is vital for the transfer of all the vitamins and minerals from our food into our cells and tissues for many health benefits.

This combination of protein, fats, and carbohydrates in a complete mini meal every 3-4 hours is the KEY to healthy weight loss.

CHAPTER 3

SETTING UP A GET IN SHAPE EXERCISE PROGRAM

When it comes to exercise, find a fitness facility that offers a variety of classes, qualified personal trainers, and great equipment. Working out in a gym is fun, social, cheerful, and motivating. You may want to check out local schools, colleges, and churches for classes or special programs. CD's and DVD's are available for working out at home and of course, there are simple pleasures like walking in your neighborhood.

The most important thing is to have fun and be consistent in whatever form of exercise you choose. The amount of exercise each person needs will vary. However, a program which features a 40– or 60-minute workout for 3-4 days per week is a great beginning. It is important to do SOMETHING every day because you will find that it will make you feel better throughout the day and sleep better at night.

Get in shape Small steps for big results

You will find that exercise does so much for you. It can reduce stress, increase strength and flexibility, give you energy, clear your head, and reduce body fat. It is the BEST way to slow down the aging process. Look for nationally certified instructors and personal trainers and ask to speak to their clients for recommendations.

Exercise including cardiovascular work and weight training will play an important role in your daily regimen. You want to do an exercise that will increase your heart rate and elevate your body temperature for 30 minutes each day. This allows the body to burn calories and reduce body fat. Exercise strengthens muscles and bones to help prevent osteoporosis.

Make an outline of a typical day of meals to note what time you eat breakfast, lunch, dinner, snacks, and what beverages are consumed. Do you eat alone or with other people, and what types of foods are you eating each meal? Make sure you include snacks as well from your favorite restaurants frequented.

The right combination of foods at each meal is critical for the development of a healthy eating plan. Everyone is different and each plan must accommodate personal preferences, schedules, and individual needs. You really do have to make time to eat! Think of your body as a computer. It only functions as good as what you enter into it. If you do not enter enough information or the wrong information, the computer will malfunction. Your body is the same! You must feed your body the right foods and enough food to keep it running at optimum levels.

Quick, low-fat meals that will stay with you for at least 3 hours are the key to preparation and success. You should look forward to your meals and not feel guilty when the hunger pains begin. Think of it as a time to fuel your body! You must eat–just the right way!

CHAPTER 4

IMPORTANCE OF REST AND SLEEP

The idea of rest and relaxation eludes many of us. Consequently, we usually do not sleep enough, making it much more difficult to function at optimal capacity the next day. Night after night, without enough quality sleep, the deprivation adds up, causing us to be unproductive and unhappy in our daylight hours. It really is amazing how quickly a good night's sleep can turn that all around.

The general recommendation is to get eight hours of sleep per night. That means, if you stay up binge-watching your favorite television show until midnight and your alarm goes off at five in the morning, you will be grossly short on sleep. We have all been there, hitting snooze and praying that work gets canceled for the day. Well, it's not going to happen, so all we can do is get the sleep we require to prepare us for the next day. A well-rested person will have little trouble getting out of bed and will sail through their day with less stress. That is a proven fact.

Get in shape Small steps for big results

Sleep is vital for your wellbeing, but according to a 2008 study by the National Sleep Foundation, the average amount of sleep an American adult gets is two hours less than it was in 1960. When you consider that adequate sleep is vital for self-discipline and health, it's a scary statistic. This chronic lack of sleep has also been cited by some researchers as one of the reasons for the rise in obesity in the same time period.

One reason for this could be that getting less than six hours of shut-eye a night impairs your impulse control. In fact, sleep deprivation has similar effects to being mildly intoxicated, and that's definitely not a good thing for your self-control. If you're regularly getting less than adequate sleep, your prefrontal cortex becomes temporarily impaired, making it much harder to resist the impulses of your lizard brain (the oldest part of the brain, or the brain stem). Your body starts to react to normal everyday stressors in a primitive fight-or-flight manner because your lizard brain is in the driving seat. Your cortisol levels rise and your willpower depletes rapidly.

Try to sleep at least 6.5 to 8 hours a night and you'll see a big difference. Eliminate all noise in your room or try to listen to Zen-like, soothing sounds. Dim the lights and drink a glass of cherry juice before going to sleep. Take a warm shower, too, if you want—so you'll easily be able to fall asleep.

Get in shape Small steps for big results

Upon waking up the next day, you'll feel like you have so much energy to do what you want. If this happens every day, it would be so good for you and your health!

If you sleep less than seven hours per night, your brain cannot do its job of maintaining itself properly. Your brain is like a self-cleaning oven. It switches on to "clean mode" while you sleep to remove all the viruses and bacteria that come in through your nose and mouth during the day. By using plaque and tangles which are made of sticky-like substances, your brain cleans, repairs, and regenerates itself. This process takes seven to nine uninterrupted hours to complete this important task correctly. But if your brain is interrupted mid-cleaning cycle, the plaque and tangles remain, and, in time, they begin to accumulate and cut off blood flow to the neurons in your brain. Without blood flow, your neurons begin to die off.

Have you ever experienced brain fog after a night of little or no sleep? This is caused by the brain's inability to regenerate correctly, leaving the sticky plaques to accumulate. Your thoughts literally cannot connect. You forget words, you stumble to remember names, and you feel depleted and confused. This is what dementia patients often experience. It is frustrating and scary. Sleep cures this problem. Let the self-cleaning process in your brain do its job.

CHAPTER 5

STRESS FREE WEIGHT LOSS

Stress can play a big role in stopping you from achieving your weight loss goals. When you implement changes slowly into your life, you dramatically increase your success. This is because you are reducing the amount of stress in your life.

Stress, apart from making you tired and anxious, can also make you gain weight and reduce the positive elements of your dedication and hard work. This is because when you are stressed, your body produces certain hormones that contribute to weight gain and can do so at a rapid pace.

Before you start introducing new habits to get in shape, it is recommended that you try and reduce as much stress as you possibly can.

There are many benefits gained from reducing stress and losing weight and everyone should take the time to enjoy them. The first thing you will notice is that your energy levels increase. You'll go from feeling sluggish one week to feeling energized and happier the next. You'll notice that it's easier to say no to unhealthy foods and yes to healthier ones, which in turn leaves your hair and skin looking and feeling great.

When you feel great about yourself, you feel much more positive towards other parts of your life, creating a better balance. Mentally and physically, you'll soon see that you become more confident about the way you look and how you deal with other people, and you'll see an increase into how much effort you put into establishing healthier habits in your daily life.

As you become healthier, you see the world in a better light. You are more likely to eat healthy in the long term, stay in shape, and take more opportunities in your social life. When you eat healthy and take the time to look after your physical health, your confidence and positivity shines through each action you make. You will find that it's easier to adopt healthier habits over time, which then increases your positivity and reduces your anxiety.

CHAPTER 6

EXERCISES TO HELP YOU GET IN SHAPE

Weighted T-Exercise

Stand with your feet slightly staggered, right foot in front of the left. Shift your weight onto the right leg and slightly bend your knee. Lift the left leg off of the ground and lower your torso until it becomes parallel with your lifted leg.

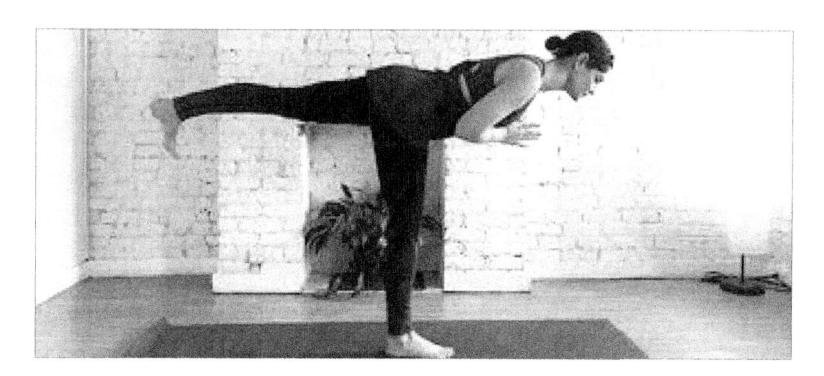

With control, lower the left leg back down to the ground and return to the starting position to finish 1 rep. Do all of your reps on one side before switching sides to finish 1 set. **Try:** 2 reps with legs holding the position 15 to 20 sec each.

Sit-ups

These are common like pushups. Of course, you have seen them done. But just in case, here is how you do it correctly: Anchor your feet firmly. Now, like bicycle crunches, you want to put your hands behind your head or across the front of your chest. Whichever is better for you. Then form a diamond shape with your arms if you go with the behind the head position or cross your arms into an X if you go with the across the chest position.

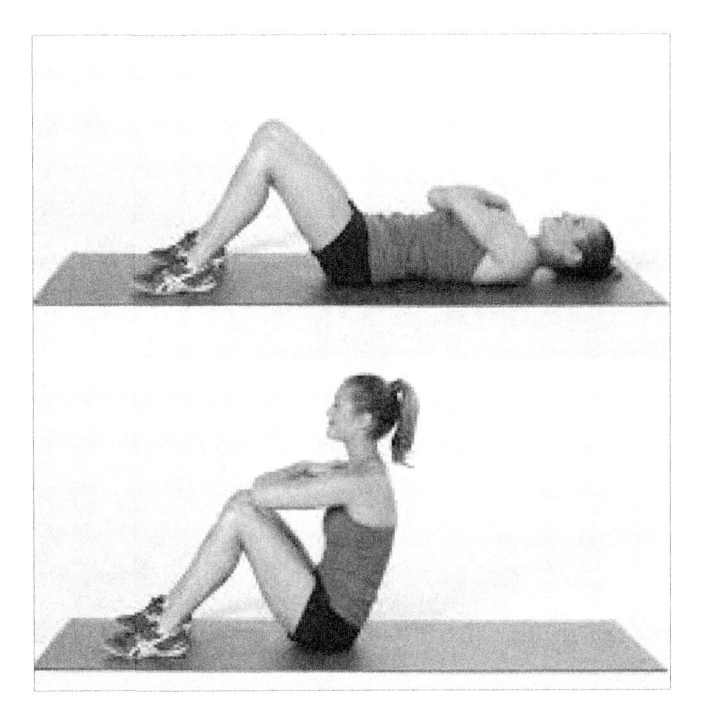

When you sit up you want to inhale; exhale when you lie back down. Speed doesn't mean that you are doing better in this exercise so take it slow and stay in control. Keep your back straight and your abdomen flexed.

Do not pull yourself up with your arms. You want to use your core muscles to do all of the work. That is the only way that it is going to work for you. The only thing you want to move is your core. The rest has to stay perfectly in position as you sit up and lower yourself back down. Don't lift your feet off the floor either.

Try: 10 reps 5 times. 10 set-ups in each rep. Take a 30 sec break in between each rep.

Dumbbell Press

First, for safety, make sure there are no other weights on the floor near the bench. If you get tired, you don't want to put the dumbbells down and accidentally smash your finger between another weight.

Start very light to assess your strength and get the feel for it. Ladies start with 10- or 15-pound dumbbells, and men start with 20-pound weights. Yes, they might seem very light but we're just assessing our strength so adjust accordingly.

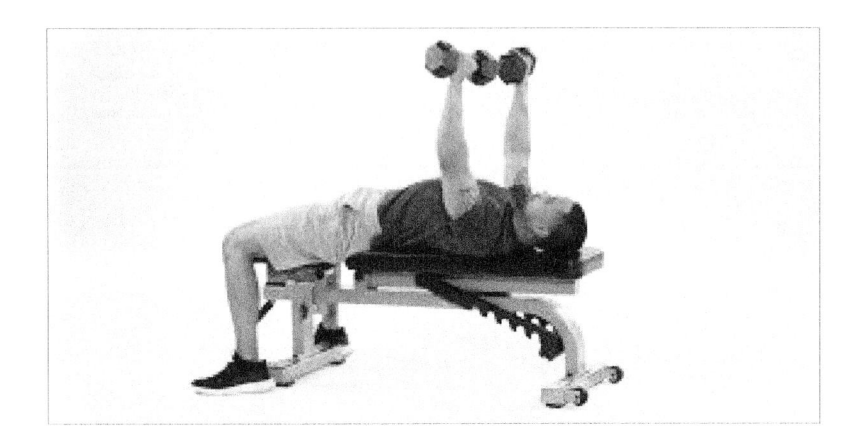

Sit on a bench with the dumbbells on your thighs, then lay back slowly and controlled while lifting the dumbbells from your thighs to your chest.

Now that you are lying flat on the bench, exhale strongly as you push the dumbbells straight up into the air. Do not lock your arms at the top; keep them just barely bent so that your muscles are working and not resting in the locked position.

Hold the weights for a second and then bring them down slowly, taking about three seconds. **Try:** 10 reps 5 times, resting in between each rep.

Hamstrings/Back

Stand with your feet together.

Bend at the waist keeping your legs completely straight (lock your knees if you need to).

Extending your arms, try to touch your toes. If this isn't a challenge for you, try to lay your palms flat on the ground in front of your toes.

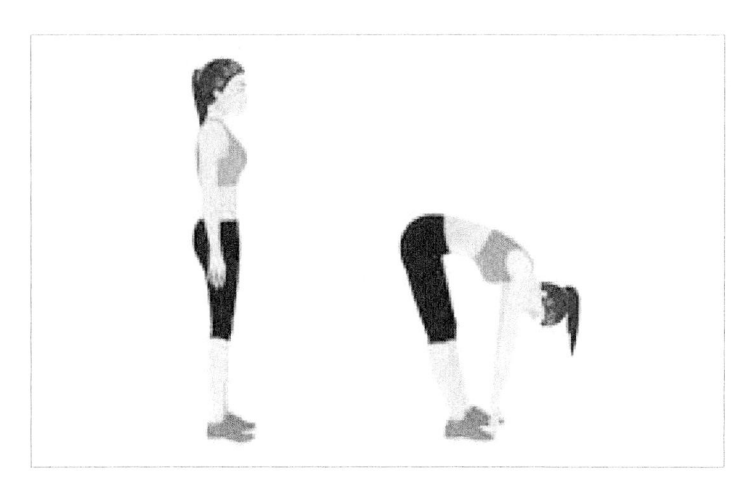

Hold this position for 15 seconds. **Try:** 3 reps at 15 seconds each.

Stability Hip Raise

Bring yourself into a plank position on your forearms with the medicine ball between your thighs. First, work to get the entire body parallel to the ground. Then, as you squeeze your thighs against the ball, press down with your forearms and lift your hips into the air.

Get in shape Small steps for big results

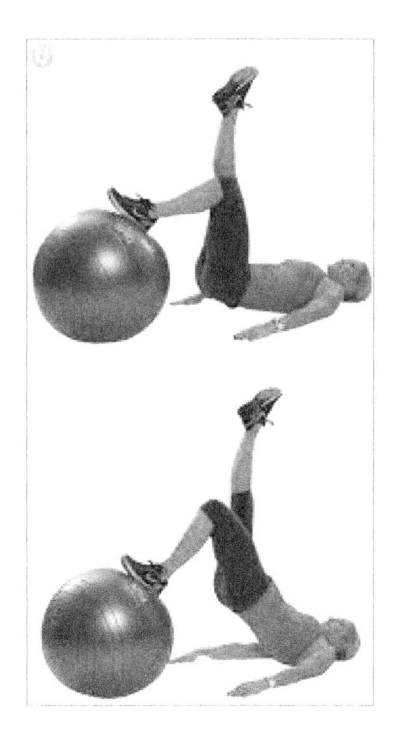

Lower slowly back to the starting position to complete 1 rep.

Try to stay in the plank position throughout the whole set with the knees and legs lifted off the ground. **Try:** 15 seconds each rep, 2 reps a peace with each leg..

Speed Walk

As the name suggests, speed walking is an ideal form of aerobic exercise that enables you to improve your cardiovascular health. The legs move quicker as the arms pump you ahead. For speed walking, you may walk at a certain pace; say a mile in 14 minutes. This is considered one of the best types of walking to help you lose weight, keep fit, and maintain a good shape–and ultimately live a healthy life.

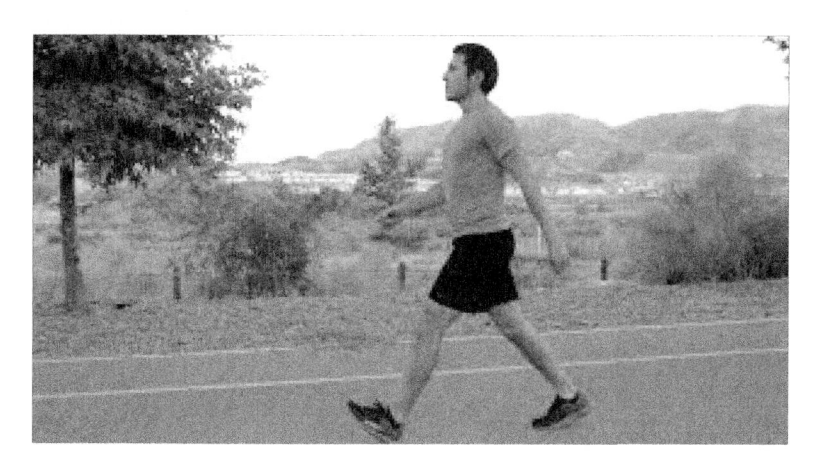

Dumbbell flyes

Hold a pair of dumbbells with your arms loosely at your sides.

Slowly extend your arms outward with the dumbbells at your sides, keeping your elbows slightly bent.

When you've raised them to shoulder height, pause briefly and then slowly lower them back to the start position.

Exhale as you lift the dumbbells.

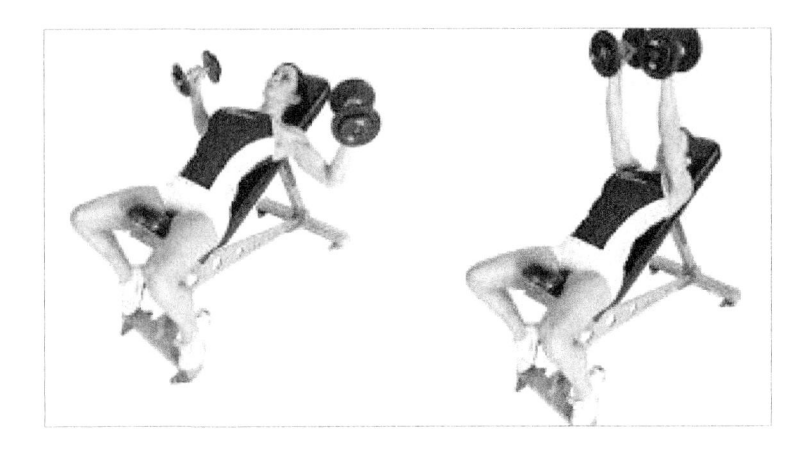

Inhale as you lower them.

Keep your elbows fixed in a stable position and slightly bent throughout the exercise.

You really want to feel this in your traps so adjust your body until you really feel the exercise target that area. **Try:** 10 reps 5 times, resting in between each rep.

Triceps Press

The companion exercise to the curl is the triceps press. This works the muscles on the back of the arm.

The tricep muscles are essential to every pushing or pressing movement you do. The dumbbell movement here is intended to enhance strength in the full range of motion for the triceps.

Begin by holding the dumbbell in your hands. Push the dumbbell overhead to arm's length, while still holding them.

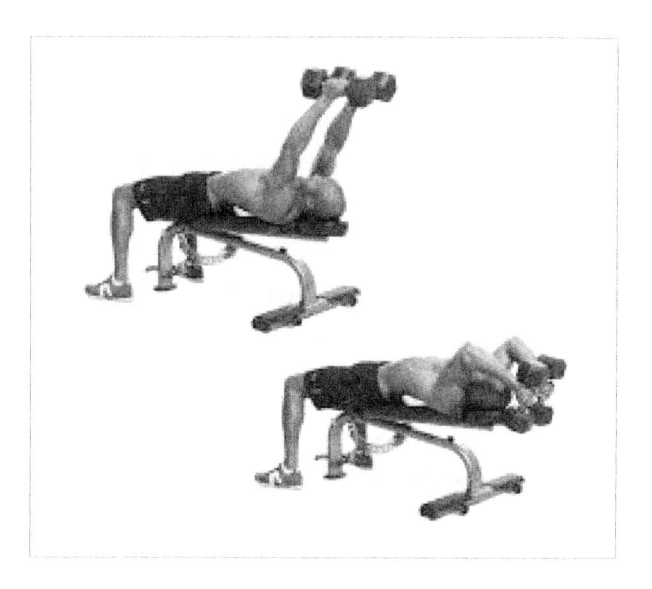

Take a deep breath and slowly lower the weight behind your head. Try to keep your elbows pointed directly upward.

Lower the weight behind your head as far as you can go without experiencing pain. Keeping the elbows pointed upward, use your triceps to push the weight back to a point where it is directly overhead.

Triceps press: starting position Triceps press: lower position

As in the curl, strict form is more important than the amount of weight you use. The purpose of this phase of training is getting your full range of motion restored. **Try:** 10 reps 5 times, resting in between each rep.

Seated Arm Stretch

Sit with your legs crossed and your back straight.

Stretch both arms up towards the sky as high as you can reach and lock your fingers together.

Continue reaching as high as possible stretching the muscles in your arms.

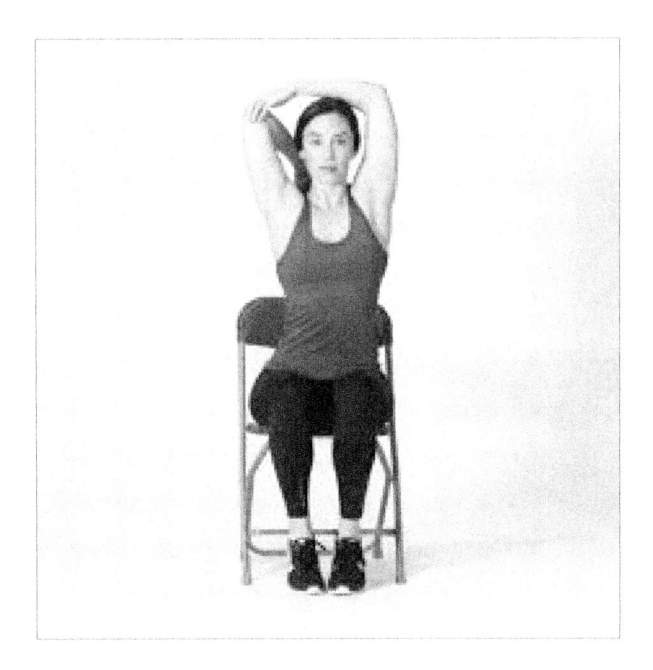

Hold

Try: 30 seconds, do this 1-2 times

Kettlebell/Dumbbell Goblet Squat

The squat is the king of body strength exercises and should be a mainstay in any conditioning program.

In reconditioning it is particularly important that you focus on restoring your full range of motion. Most people who reach age 50 will have lost a lot of flexibility and strength in squatting motions.

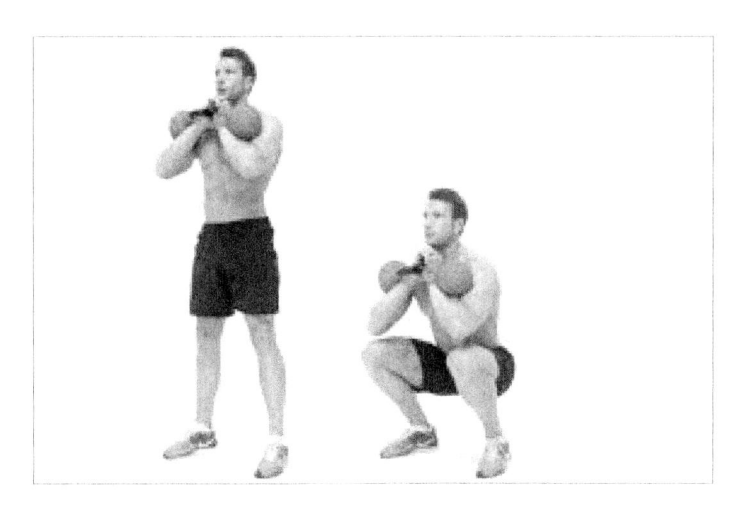

If you had problems with your knees or back when doing the unweighted squat, you should continue to work without weights until you can easily perform squats.

Leg press or leg extension machines are NOT a proxy for doing free standing squats. Machine lifts will rob you of your ability to balance and control weights in space. In short, the machine will suck all the athletic performance out of any lift.

Begin by standing upright with your feet slightly wider than shoulder width. You will be holding a kettlebell (or dumbbell) just below your chin. Hold the kettlebell by each side of the handle or hold a dumbbell by one end.

Keep your head facing forward and your chest up and out. In a smooth motion, sit down and back as if you were sitting onto an imaginary chair. Lower down until your thighs are parallel to the floor.

Be sure to keep your knees over your ankles for proper position. Press your weight into your heels. Push through your heels to bring your body back up to the standing position. **Try:** 10 reps 5 times, resting in between each rep.

Leg Raise

Begin by lying on your back on the floor. Place your hands at your sides. Take a deep breath and hold it. Keeping your legs straight, raise one leg off the floor until it's elevated to a 45-degree angle and hold it until you feel the burn.

Lower your legs back gently to the starting position on the floor and release your breath.

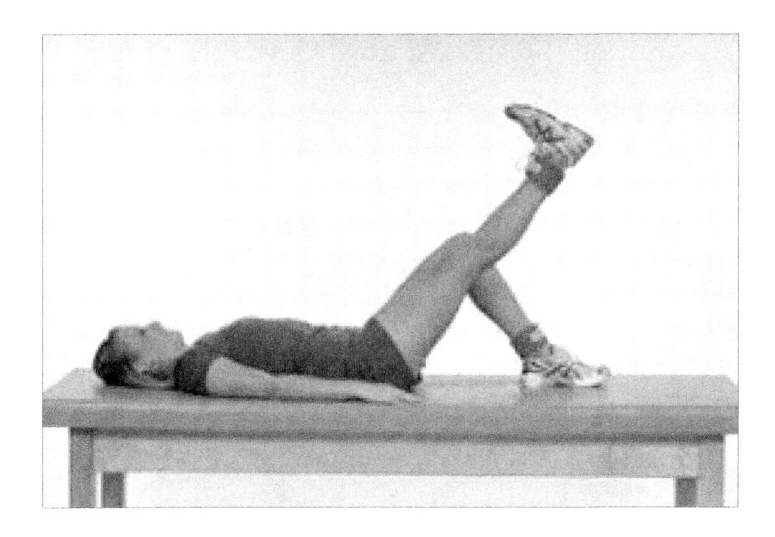

If this exercise is too difficult with straight legs, bend your knees slightly so that you can do the required number of reps.

Don't bounce your feet off the floor when you are doing reps. Start each repetition from a dead stop. **Try:** 10 reps 5 times, 5 with each leg resting in between each rep.

One Arm Rowing

Begin by placing your right knee on a bench. Bend over and place your right hand on the bench. Your left foot should be on the floor.

Take a dumbbell at arm's length in your left hand. Take a deep breath and pull the dumbbell up to your waist using your back muscles (lats) to do the lifting. When the dumbbell is at your waist, release your breath and slowly lower the weight back to the starting position.

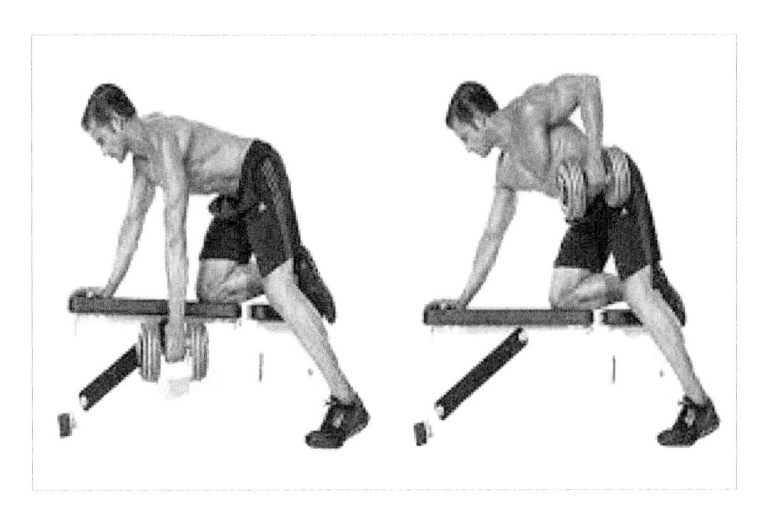

Pull the dumbbell up to your waist in a smooth motion. Make your lat muscles do all the work. Don't jerk the weight or use your body to generate momentum.

Use a relatively heavy weight. **TRY:** 4 reps 2 times each arm. That's 10 each arm with this exercise.

One hand dumbbell row: starting and top position

American Swing

Stand with your feet wide, holding the kettlebell with both hands in between your legs. Bend your knees slightly but keep your back straight. Swing the kettlebell up all the way over your head with straight arms. As you do so, straighten the legs and thrust the hips forward. Keep your heels on the ground the entire time, pushing down into the ground with them for more power.

Return to the starting position to finish 1 rep.

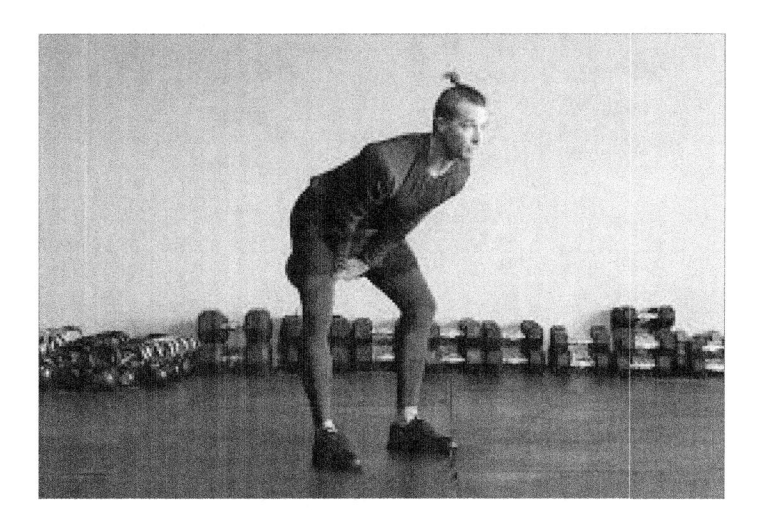

Note: The swings should be done consecutively without stopping so that you work with the momentum of the weight. Be careful to not stop abruptly mid-swing – come to a stop slowly after finishing your reps. **Try:** 10 reps 5 times, resting in between each rep.

Dumbbell Pushup Pulls

In order to perform this exercise, you will need dumbbells of some type. The heavier the weight, the more difficult the exercise.

Place two dumbbells on the ground about shoulder-width apart.

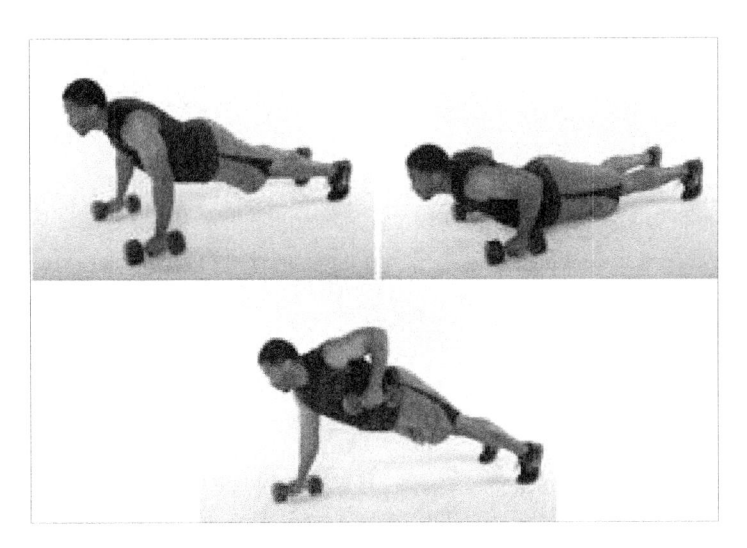

Get into a normal pushup position but instead of placing your hands flat on the floor, grip the dumbbells with each hand. The dumbbells should be laid lengthwise so that when you grip them, your palms are facing each other.

Perform the push up, lowering yourself as far as you can go.

When you return to the start position, raise the dumbbell in your right hand as far up as you can (bending at the elbow) until the dumbbell touches your chest, and then return it to the ground.

Repeat with another pushup, and then raise the left dumbbell.

Repeat, alternating each side for the duration of the set.

Inhale as you lower your body, and then slowly start to exhale as you raise yourself back up to the start position. Continue to exhale as you raise the dumbbell.

Next, instead of stopping when you raise the dumbbell to your chest, rotate your body away from the dumbbell and continue raising it to the sky until your arm is straight.

Try: 30 seconds, continuous, 30 seconds rest. Do 3 sets. Increase either the weight of the dumbbells or the time per set (or both) as you improve.

Leg Raise Bridge

Lie down flat on an exercise mat or whatever you use and keep your arms by your sides, knees bent.

Keep your feet flat on the floor.

Lift your left leg off the ground and raise your hips simultaneously by pushing off your right heel.

Keep your hips in a straight line with your chest (diagonal).

Get in shape Small steps for big results

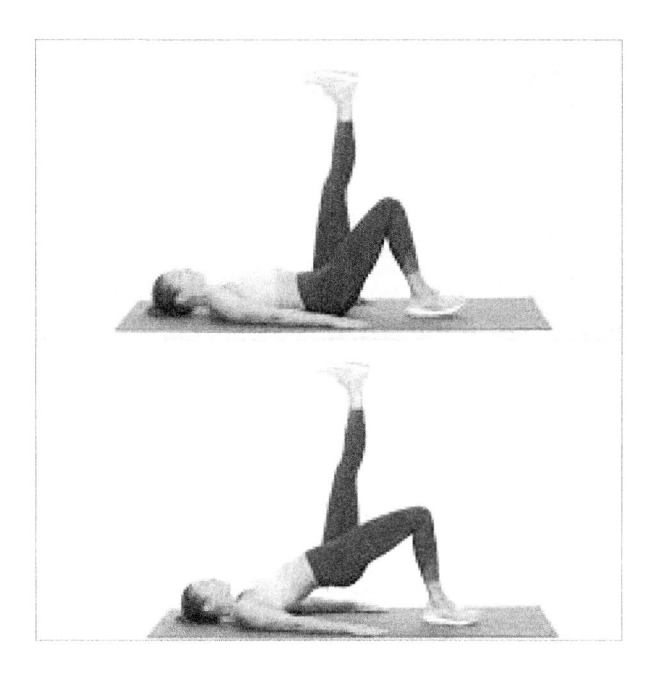

Hold this posture for a few seconds and lower your hips.

Repeat the same process with the other leg.

Exhale when you raise the hips.

Make sure your glutes and abs remain tight throughout the process.

Keep your upper body in a comfortable and neutral posture.

Try: Performing 3 sets of 8 to 12 reps for each leg.

Abdominal Plank

Building your core strength is one of the most important things you can do for having good health and quality of life. Core strength is critical for preventing chronic conditions such as back pain, leg pain, and knee pain from emerging as you age.

You will need a timer for this exercise as you will be doing it for a specific number of seconds. An inexpensive stopwatch will work well, or the second hand on any available clock. There are many options.

Begin by getting on the floor as if you were going to do push ups. Rest your weight on your forearms and your toes. Raise your hips up until all your weight is resting on your forearms and toes. Keep your back straight and don't allow your rear end to go up in the air.

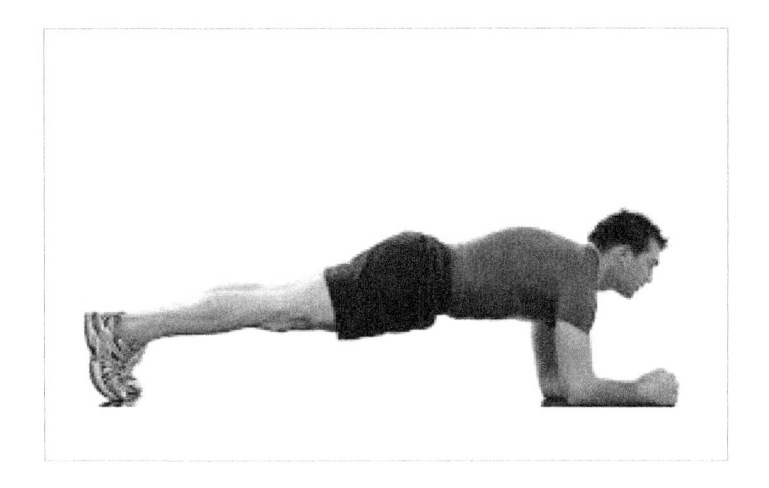

You should hold the position shown in the photo for 10-30 seconds. Work up to the point where you can hold the plank position for at least 30 seconds each time.

That concludes the resistance training part of the workout. Now for the aerobics.

Lunge Reach Stretch

Get into the lunge position keeping your body in a straight line from head to toe.

Lead with your left foot and place your right hand on the floor next to your right foot.

Stretch with your left hand towards the ceiling rotating your body slightly.

Get in shape Small steps for big results

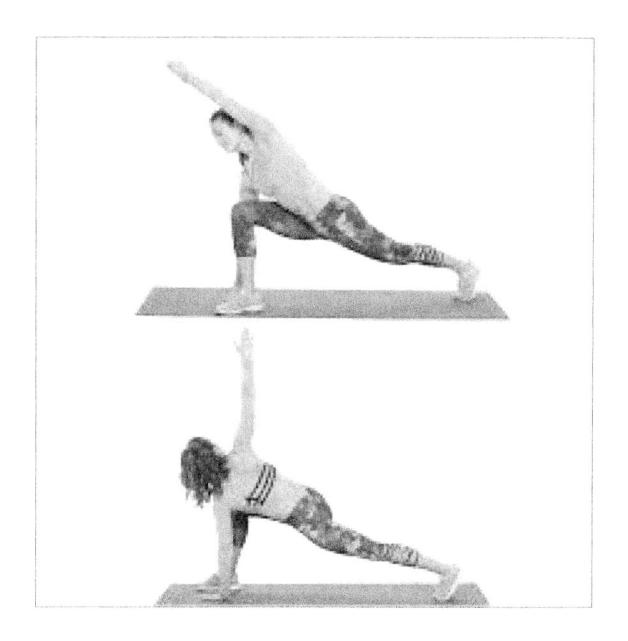

Hold, and then switch sides.

Try: 30 seconds each side at least 2 times

<u>Single Leg Calf Raise</u>

Follow the same instructions as the standing calf raise (see exercise 1) but implement the variations in the following steps.

There are two ways to do this exercise:

Lift your right foot off the ground and raise it behind you, bending at the knee until your leg is at a 90-degree angle (shin parallel to the ground behind you).

Get in shape Small steps for big results

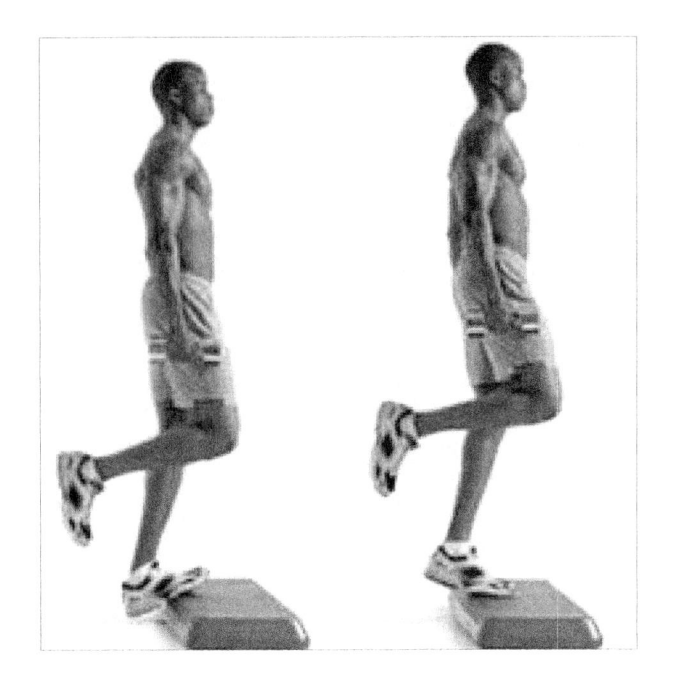

OR

The harder way: raise your knee in front of you until your thigh is parallel to the ground (leg at a 90-degree angle raised in front of you–see picture)

Raise up onto the ball of your left foot, which is planted on the ground and squeeze your calf muscle.

Lower yourself as far as you can, arching your foot downward before repeating.

Exhale as you rise onto the balls of your feet and squeeze your calf muscle. Inhale as you lower yourself back down. **Try:** 30 seconds each leg at least 2 times

Mountain Runners

Starting in a plank position, move your right knee toward your chest, and hold. After that, spot your foot in the plank position. Bring your left knee into your chest. Keep your tummy muscles pulled in. **Try:** for 40 seconds and then rest for 10 seconds.

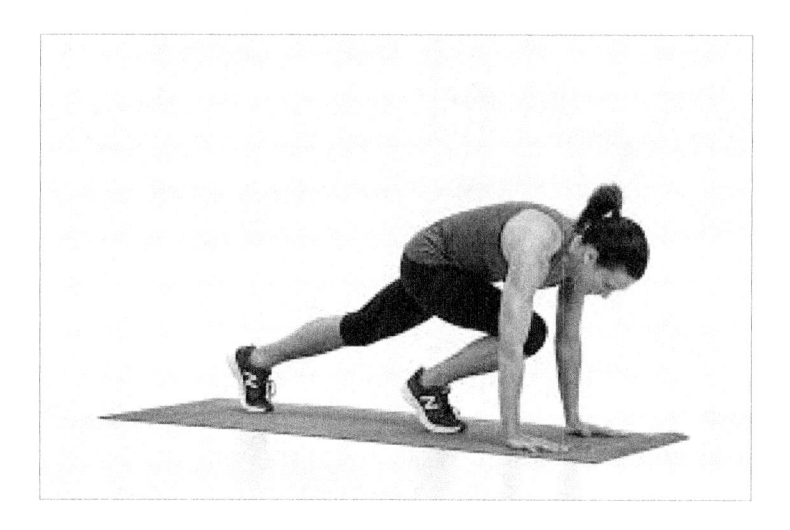

Glute Lift

Lie flat on the floor on your back and keep your hands at your sides and knees bent.

Slowly lift your butt off the floor keeping your shoulders on the ground.

Stay in this position for a few seconds but remember when you lift your butt your body should remain in a straight line.

Flex your glutes and really strain and push up with your butt.

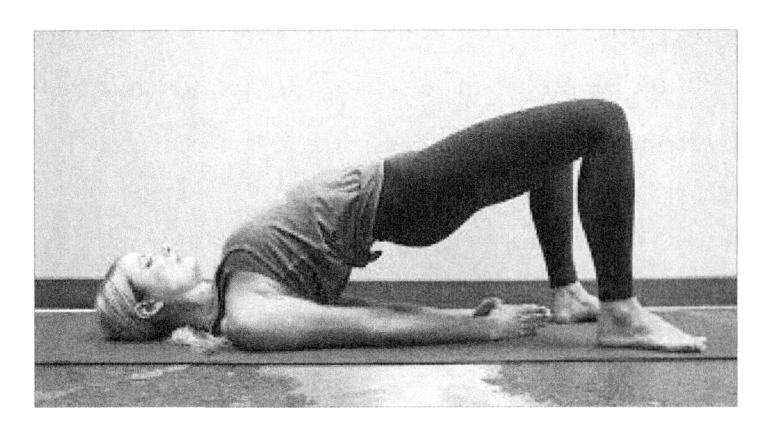

Come back to the starting position and repeat.

Exhale as you lift your butt off the ground.

Inhale as you go back to the starting position.

Try: At least 2 to 3 sets of 10 reps and increase the reps when you get enough strength.

Bicycle crunches

Cycling is one of the best cardio exercises. This leaves little room for surprise when I tell you that bicycle crunches are fantastic for weight loss. It is fairly easy to do and brings great results when done correctly.

How to do them: Start by lying down on the floor on your back. Now pretend that you are lounging on the beach with your hands under your head for support. Your arms should make a sort of diamond shape.

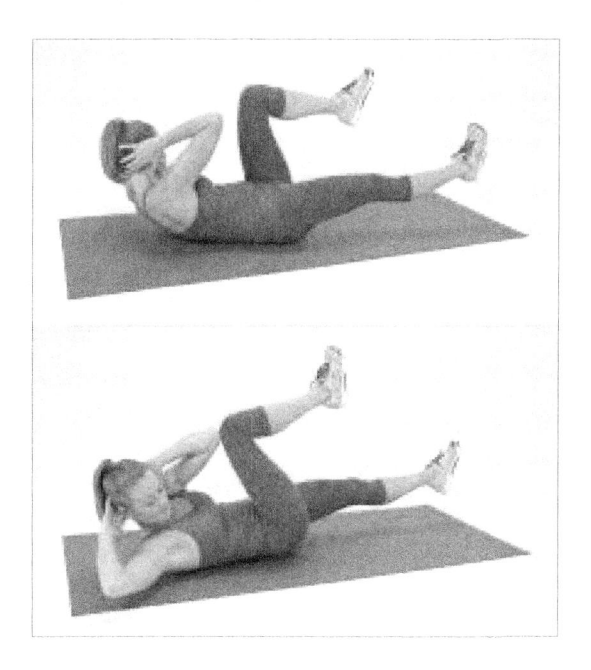

Start pedaling! Pretend that you are on a bicycle and you are trying to win the race! Bring one knee up to your chest while stretching the other one straight. Don't let the straight leg touch the ground. If you are pulling up your left knee, touch your left knee with your right elbow and vice versa. Twist as far as you have to, to touch those knees and elbows.

Start slow and leave your arms and back firmly on the ground. Just pedal for a while to get used to it and to find the right rhythm you want to go at. When you are feeling comfortable enough, you can go ahead and add the elbows to knees motion. Remember to clench those abdomen muscles to get the full effect.

Try: 20 knee to elbow touches in a rep at least 2 times. Take a break in between.

Side Crunch

Lie on your side with your body rotated slightly inward towards your stomach.

Move your upper body and legs inward keeping both straight until your body forms a 45-degree angle.

Prop your upper body up slightly on your elbow and place your other hand behind your head with your elbow bent.

Keep your feet together and legs as straight as possible.

Crunch sideways, lifting your right leg up and curling your upper body up, trying to reach your feet with your elbow.

Lower your leg back to the starting position but do not let it touch the other until the set has been completed. Repeat.

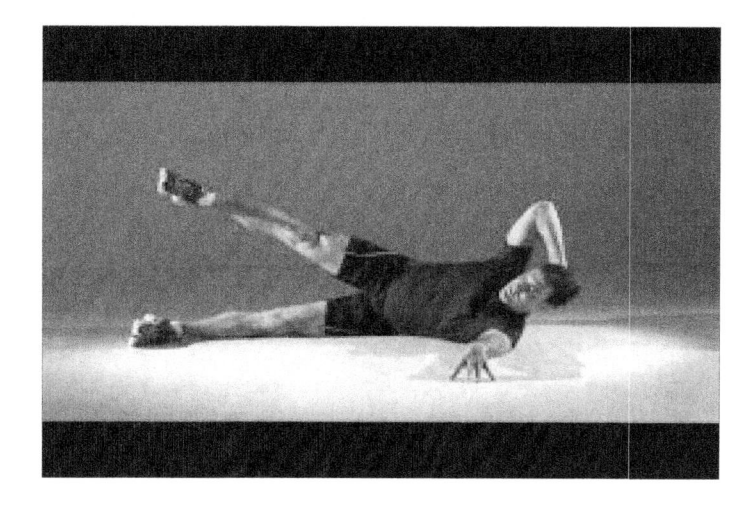

After the set is completed, roll onto your other side and do the exercise from that side.

Exhale as you raise your legs and inhale as you lower them.

Try: 15 reps on your left and 15 on your right. Do 3 sets per side.

Side Plank

Get into pushup position and lower yourself onto your elbows (with your whole body off the ground).

Roll onto your left side so you are supported by your left elbow. Stretch your right arm straight up to the ceiling for balance.

Keep your body as straight as possible and clench your core.

Get in shape Small steps for big results

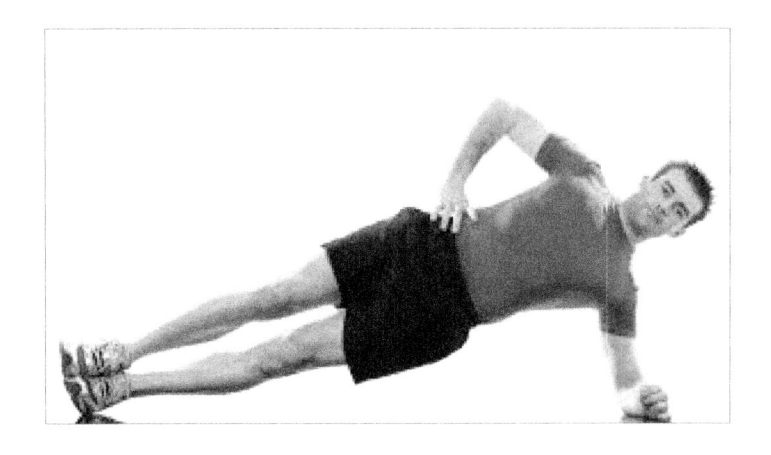

Hold for the duration of the set. Then go back to the pushup position and rotate to your other side, then repeat.

This is a continuous burn, so just take controlled deep breaths throughout. Keep your breaths consistent and slow.

Try: 15 sec on your left and 15 on your right. Do at least twice per side.

Plank Ups

Start in the plank position and keep your hands straight under your shoulders, resting on your elbows. Be sure to keep your back straight.

Your toes should touch the floor. Squeeze your glutes to stabilize your body.

Keep your legs straight and your hands should remain in a line.

Hold the plank position for 15-20 seconds, then raise up onto your palms, fully extending your arms and flex your core. Hold that position for 10 seconds and then return back onto your elbows for the plank position.

Continue repeating for the indicated set.

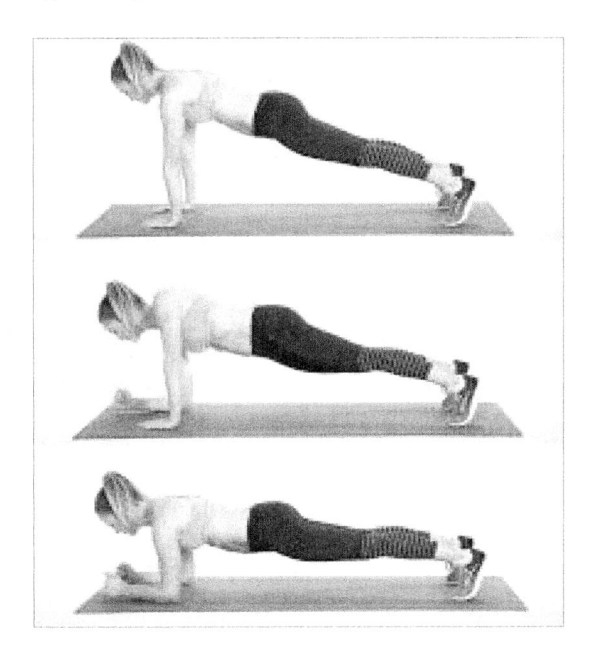

Take continuous measured breaths all the way through.

Throughout the exercise, keep your spine, head, and neck in a straight line.

If you are a beginner, first practice elbow planks and strengthen your core.

Get in shape Small steps for big results

Try: this exercise continuously for 2 minutes, then take a 30 second rest. Do 2-3 sets.

Jump squats

These are just like normal squats but with a little bit extra spice. These squats are the big sister of normal squats and can really work a person's body. Once the normal squat is perfected, this is the next step to those perfectly toned glutes and thighs.

How to do them: Just like normal squats, you want to keep your feet shoulder-width apart. Now do a squat like you would begin a regular one but instead of coming back up to stand in your original position, you are going to push yourself off the floor and jump straight up in the air. When you land, you want to move back into that squat position. Your goal is to either be in the squat position, or in the air. You want to land as quietly as possible.

Get in shape Small steps for big results

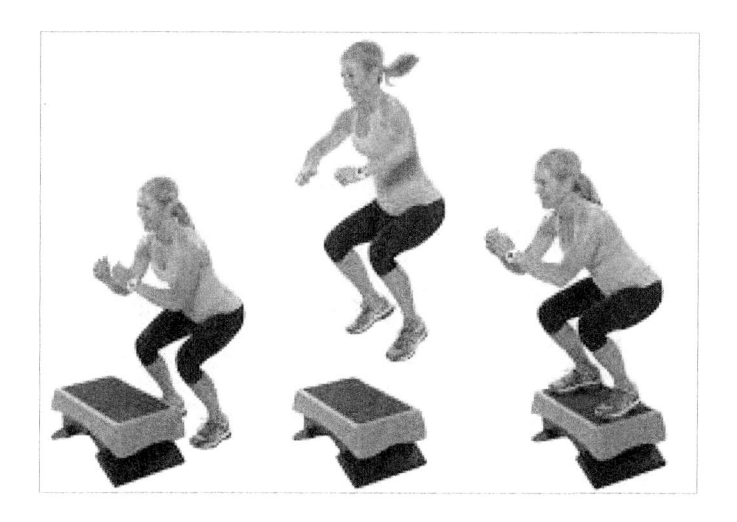

When jumping, keep your arms straight out above your head and return them in their bent position when you are on the floor again.

Try: 10 reps 5 times, resting in between each rep.

CHAPTER 7

TIPS TO GET MOTIVATED

Journals and calendars are your friends

Keeping track of your progress is important when you are exercising. Logging your progress in a journal is great motivation. Why? Because whenever you feel like giving up, you go back to the journals and have a look at where you started and where you are now. Sometimes that is the only motivation a person needs. Keeping track of progress on a calendar keeps it in clear view and the same goes for your goals. Calendars are also great for goal setting.

Get rid of negativity

Now, walk around your house and shove all of the negativity into a trash bag. Literally, take a plastic bag and walk through your house. If the negatives are invisible, then imagine them being picked from the air and shoved into the trash bag. The imagination is a wonderful thing, and in this way, you can convince your brain that there is no negativity around you anymore. This means that you can now focus solely on the positive.

Surround yourself with motivation

Everything around you should motivate you. The world is a beautiful place full of things that need accomplishing and butts that need kicking. Surround yourself with people that support you and motivate you to get up and do things. Get rid of the downers. Those people don't end up accomplishing much in life and they won't help you either.

Have a goal in mind

Set milestones and goals. For example, you might want to try five sit-ups before you do ten. Five is your first milestone and you want to achieve that by the end of the week. Think small at first. Do one week, even one day at a time. Planning months ahead can get overwhelming really fast, surely ending up in failure.

Group activities aren't always bad

You need to get a community going. Find people with the same dreams that share the same obstacles and troubles. If you are a single mom, there are a hundred more in the neighborhood that struggle with raising their kids and being adults at the same time. They also struggle with losing the weight that they still blame on their pregnancy years before. Surround yourself with people who know where you are coming from and work together to reach your goals. Those people also tend to check in on your progress, providing some accountability. Also, there is a little competitor in all of us. Let that person show.

Schedules

Schedule time to work out and stick to it. It's easy to schedule a time to exercise, but then you remember the pie in the oven, or that your son needs a costume for his play. There is always something to do and it's always more important than exercising. Eventually, when you get to the time of day that you need to work out, your body will let you know. It will crave it. Create a schedule that suits you best and during that time period, nothing is coming into your bubble. Everything else can wait.

Tell yourself that working out is fun!

You have to tell yourself that this is a good thing and although you might not enjoy the exercise, you will enjoy the endorphins and eventually, the results. That makes working out fun and worth it. Ban all negativities toward exercising and replace them with good vibes. Tiptoe around the fact that you do not enjoy it. Soon enough, it will become a part of your routine, just like brushing your teeth.

Don't fight the addiction

It's common for a person to become addicted to post-workout hormones. It makes you feel happy and energized and for some reason, people tend to fight it. The only thing I can tell you is, don't. Don't fight the addiction. This is a good kind of addiction that will improve your quality of life instead of ruining it. This is a good kind of addiction so embrace it. Take it like you would take a vitamin tablet, knowing that it's good for you. Give in to the addiction when you feel like working out–even if it's only a few squats.

Playlists and audiobooks

Know that you have set audiobooks for your workouts. They have to be binge worthy and addictive. They have to seduce you into working out.

Everything's a competition

Compete with your yesterday's self, your exercise buddy, or even the set list of exercises you have. If you do one extra sit-up, that means that you have won, and the satisfaction is your prize. If you are working out in a group, you can either secretly compete or create a competition among yourselves. It will not only motivate you, but you will motivate others too and that is a great person to be–the motivator.

Television

Plan your workouts around your favorite shows. Either use it as a reward system to motivate yourself to workout, or workout while watching your shows. That way you will associate exercise with a good time rather than begrudgingly doing it on your own in boredom. If you start your day with a run, at least you know your day can't get any worse.

Get in shape Small steps for big results

Start small

The biggest mistake people do is start too big. You can't, it's impossible. Does a toddler walk before they crawl? No, so why do you want to do that? If you are not used to exercise, chances are that your body is going to feel the slightest extra movements in a day and that is good. You want to at least feel like you exercised but not to the point where you can't walk. People want to start big to prove a point and that is stupid. Not only do you set yourself up for failure, you also create a mammoth task that you will be afraid of tackling.

Remember why you are doing it

This right here is why setting goals is so important. You need to keep in mind the reason behind why you are doing it and then use it as fuel. If you are doing it for your health, keep that in mind. If you are doing it to lose weight, maybe your goal weight should be written somewhere or stuck to the fridge. Maybe a photo of your dream body should be with it.

Motivate others

You can't motivate a person to do something if you're not going to do it yourself. Practice what you preach, buddy. This is great for forcing yourself to burn those calories and stay motivated. You now have an image to keep up and the only way that you are going to do that is by exercising.

Post-workout analysis

Write down what you are feeling after you have had your workout. It's often easy to forget the good when you are trying to convince yourself to get out of bed and get to working out. The hardest part is getting started and reading how you feel afterwards will remind you about the great effect that exercise has on your mind and body.

CHAPTER 8

MEASURE YOUR PROGRESS

This is another important point you have to keep in mind. As a weight reduction strategy, it becomes extremely important to be mindful of the number of pounds which you are losing. If you don't keep track of the amount of weight you are losing, things will not work out the right way for you.

This is the reason you are requested to measure the progress in an apt manner. Losing weight is not a cakewalk. Belly fat in particular can be persistent as this fat tends to get accumulated in between the visceral organs.

This is why you need to be mindful of the progress you are making. Before you start a workout session, you need to record your weight. One common mistake which a lot of people make is that they base their belly fat reduction progress chart merely on the basis of weight. This is a wrong parameter to choose because sometimes you lose body fat, but this will not be proportional to your weight count.

A loss of body fat percentage is more desired because when you can attain the perfect body fat percentage your body will have a proportionate size which is definitely more desirable. When you lose body fat, you have to be sure that you do not end up losing all your muscles as this is only going to cause problems for you.

This is why you will need different techniques for the sake of measuring how far you have progressed. When you are working on weight loss methods, you will need some of the best regimes. As we have already mentioned the kind of diet and exercise training you need to carry out, we will now instruct you regarding how you can keep track of your progress.

Take Periodic Photos

It is important to take pictures of your body from different angles. Pictures give an insight, if not an accurate depiction of your physical size and shape. Sometimes, your weighing scale may show absolutely no change and too many people get disappointed by the lack of results and lose hope in their training.

There are different things you need to know in this regard. First of all, visceral fat is difficult to lose, and this is why it is going to require more time and effort. Do not expect to see immediate results. You have to be patient enough to keep working out for the long haul.

If not for anything else, do it for the photos. Do it for the exercise photos, the post-workout photos, and the photos you'll be able to take without being ashamed of your body. Be the Instagrammer that you always wanted to be. Do it for the followers, if not for yourself. The photos are a great motivator to some people and although it might seem stupid, it works. You might start out doing it for other people but once the bug has bitten you, you will forget about them soon enough.

If you follow the perfect diet chart and you are also spending enough time for the different workout sessions, it will surely bring a difference to the way you look. Belly fat tends to make your body disproportionate and when you are taking pictures, you should try and analyze whether or not you have managed to attain the perfect figure.

Measure Your Body Parts

Another thing which you should do is ensure that you take different measurements. Measure the thickness of your belly region, note down your waistline, your biceps, thighs, and likewise. Make it a point to write down all these readings because every time you sit down to measure them again, you can compare it with the previous measure to see the changes. Sometimes, a very slight change may not lead to substantial change in weight; however, even if you manage to shrink your waistline marginally, that is a victory in itself.

Obviously, apart from these two tracking methods, you should always make it a point to write down what the weighing scale says. That is always an important way to analyze!

When you keep track of the measurements and they reflect a positive change, I would ask you to continue with your workout. Do not get complacent and do not give up on your training either. You will have to consistently keep on working so that you can have the body shape you desire.

What If the Results Are Not Productive?

In the rare case that your body shows absolutely no signs of improvement, you may wonder what you should do. The answer lies in diagnosing your fault. Sure enough, there must be something you may be doing wrong. Before coming to a conclusion that your body is not showing any signs of improvement, you need to continue with the exercising and dieting regime for a minimum period of one month.

If there is absolutely no positive change in a span of one month, you need to sit back and analyze what steps you are missing. Try and take things one day at a time and make it a point to plan the perfect diet chart. You must eat according to the chart. After a couple of weeks, you can start with slight cardio, keeping the diet chart the same. Then, move on to advanced exercises and keep following them.

Try and push your body a little more each day and this time, surely you will begin to find the right results in front of you. When you are motivated enough and you keep on pushing your body, you are bound to lose belly fat. The record of your progress should serve as the motivation which will inspire you to attain the perfect figure.

CHAPTER 9

ACHIEVING AMAZING RESULTS

If you're struggling with your program and wondering how you can be successful, there are a few things that you need to do. Our body has to adjust to new eating plans and rigorous exercise. You may struggle a bit to reach your goals. This is normal and it shouldn't hold you back. Here's how you can ensure that you're successful.

Work at it Each Day

You should be prepared each day to do what it takes to get in shape. You should have meal plans ready to go and you should be ready to fit in some sort of activity, even if it's just 15 minutes. The more you prepare for getting in shape each day, the better off you're going to be. Make sure you write things down and you can use gadgets to track calories, number of steps you have taken, and so on. This should be a part of your daily routine by the end of your seven days.

Don't Quit

You can't quit when you have just begun. Once you lay down the foundation, you'll see just how easy the process starts to be. You'll begin to feel better because you're eating well. You'll have fewer cravings for bad foods and you will be getting stronger because you're beginning to exercise more often. Don't sabotage yourself by quitting–you have to keep going.

Don't Allow Failure to Win

If you fail and don't do what is required one day or eat foods that you shouldn't eat, you can't allow this to sabotage you. It's okay to fail because we have all done it when it comes to diet and exercise. All you do is pick yourself up again and get back on track. Your new lifestyle isn't gone for good because you ate cheesecake the night before. In fact, every so often you should indulge a bit because we are all human. If you stick to a 90 percent healthy lifestyle and only indulge every so often, you're still going to do fine.

It's in the Mind

Getting in shape is very much a mental process so once you overcome this fact, there's no limit to what you can achieve, your mind begins to look at it differently. We all have it inside of ourselves to get in shape, and you're one of these people. A positive attitude goes a long way towards your success and once you are positive, you'll see the results start to show up. The best thing you can do is to start now. Once you make this commitment, there's nothing that will stand in your way. A healthy lifestyle and a good body are easier to achieve than you realize. It's there waiting for you so go out right now and make it happen.

<u>Change It Up</u>

You want to vary the intervals that you do. If you perform the same routine over and over, your body will quickly get used to it. You should have several routines in place that you can alternate with. This will force the body to work hard and in turn, you'll burn more calories with each exercise session. You should also introduce new exercises from time to time to challenge the muscles in new ways. This will increase the amount of fat you burn even more. The muscles need a good challenge to keep growing and you'll break through those plateaus that can hold you back.

Don't Forget a Rest Day

Intervals work well but you should have at least one full rest day. The entire body needs to recover from intense exercise so make sure you have one rest day during the week.

The power of "a plan"

When people have no plan, they will simply be drifting. Daily circumstances will push them one way one day and another direction the next. Life just "happens" is what they say.

But… YOU have a plan. Your exercise and nutrition plan are in this book.

Every month you will be using this plan to master more skills for getting fit.

How you go about **Doing** those things is determined by your mindset and motivation.

It is easy to make plans, and then ignore them. That is what a lot of people do.

You must assert that you are in control of what goes on in your life. To get in shape you must assert control over your exercise and nutrition regimen.

You must recommit every day that you will follow the exercise and nutrition program in this book.

The Power of Persistence

Being persistent is an overwhelming determinate of success in virtually any endeavor. It is the only way you will be able to find out how successful **You** can be at any given undertaking.

Talent and other innate gifts do play some role in how good you eventually become. The most important thing is for you to understand that you will only realize your full potential by working persistently at a task. In this course, you have no idea how successful you can be until you do the work!!! This program is about realizing your unique potential. Understand that at the start, you have no idea how successful you can be. Embrace the growth mindset. In the real world you never really know what you can do until you work at it!

Positive Energy

Taking on a new challenge will require the best effort you can muster. One of the most important conditions for putting out your best effort will be lots of positive energy.

Get in shape Small steps for big results

The energy will come from yourself and your attitude, and from those around you.

You begin every day with a "can do" attitude and get excited about your training and what you are going to accomplish. You feel the power of your own enthusiasm propelling you to make changes and do the things you know are needed.

Positive energy is contagious. When you dive into a task with positive enthusiasm, it energizes those around you to feel good and do their best.

Positive energy will lift you up and move you ahead. Negative energy will do just the opposite.

Negative energy feels like it sucks the air out of a room. Tasks that may have seemed a little difficult now become impossible.

Having a positive attitude can make hard work seem enjoyable. It helps you surge forward and embrace the next challenge.

A negative attitude can do just the opposite. It can stop you in your tracks before you even get started. Negativity hangs in the air like a bad smell and can undercut everything you try to do.

Being around negative people can drain your energy quickly. For them, life appears to be a trudge from one bad experience to another. They find fault with everything. They will assure you that trying to get in good condition is going to fail.

You should stay as far away from these people as possible. They will do nothing but suck the energy out of you. They are the last people you want to be around when you are trying to do something difficult.

Hang out with people who are positive and enthusiastic, particularly about your desire to get back in good condition. Their positive energy will multiply your energy.

Take Action

If someone delays acting, the chances are that they won't do anything. Procrastination becomes the normal way of life.

Many have good intentions. But they avoid acting. The longer they put off taking action the less likely it is that they will ever DO something.

High Achievement

Being a high achiever means that you may routinely place a lot of extreme expectations on yourself. It is likely that "doing a great job" is one of the ways you received a lot of approval and recognition throughout your life. This approval may have come from parents, family, co-workers, etc. In short, you were "proving yourself."

It is possible that by you being driven may still be a means of trying to prove yourself. If you recognize this, and drop the emotional overhead, you will probably do just as good of a job, but feel some satisfaction in your accomplishment.

Discipline

You are committed to getting in shape, but how do you get yourself to do what is necessary, particularly when you may not want to do something at a specific time.

The word "discipline" comes to mind. This means doing something you know you should even though your body may not want to. The real successes in life come from having the discipline to do something that may not be appealing at first.

You have exercised discipline in your life before, probably many times. If you built a successful career, the early work was not easy, and often not fun. If you mastered a difficult subject in school, you probably had to endure many hours of difficult study. If you learned to play a musical instrument, you had to do a lot of practice when you were starting out.

Getting in shape is no different. In the beginning, some parts of the experience may be difficult for you and you will have to use discipline to keep on course.

The good news is that the longer you stick with an exercise program, the more enjoyable it becomes!

CHAPTER 10

HOW TO STAY IN SHAPE FOREVER

Keeping your weight down requires losing it slowly and steadily, and most of all, being consistent with your Eat Right Schedule and Workout Program. After making some simple changes in food choices and adding consistent exercise, most of you will lose approximately 3-4 pounds the first week. Then, a weight loss of approximately 1 pound per week can be expected. It is important to do some sort of exercise each day, whether it is weight training, taking a Yoga, Pilates, or Aerobics class, or simply walking. Exercise is critical. Think about this formula:

Eating Right + Exercise = Good Shape

Successful eaters CHEAT – plan a cheat day! It means you can choose a day to eat whatever you want at every meal and simply return to your regular healthy eating habits the very next day. Be warned! Cheating on a decadent meal, for example, will make the body rebel. No matter how wonderful the food tastes going down, once the body has adjusted to eating with the proper balance of good healthy food, the shock of those excess calories, fat, and sugar will be difficult to tolerate.

If it is not a cheat day, and the need for something forbidden is desired, treat yourself to a low-fat version or instead of eating a fattening food, purchase a new workout outfit. Looking good and feeling good when you exercise makes it more fun! Learn to treat yourself without using food. Find a special place to alleviate stress. Seek surroundings that are peaceful and beautiful for you. Take time to be pampered.

There is so much pressure on women to look like the women who grace the fashion magazines and are in the endless array of infomercials and television shows. Have you asked yourself – how do they do it? How do they stay slim and fit? It takes more than scheduling workouts at the gym and gulping down a mug of coffee on the way to work. That will not sustain you for very long.

Here are some suggestions for staying fit and healthy at the same time:

- Stick to your routine– this means finding foods that work for you and keep you full without increasing your waistline. You have to take the guesswork out of eating your meals, especially breakfast and lunch. It might be egg whites scrambled with vegetables every morning and a grilled chicken salad for lunch – EVERY DAY! You might change the ingredients just a bit by making an omelet instead or substituting salmon for grilled chicken. Develop a routine that makes eating right a HABIT rather than a daily battle.

- Eat something before going to a party or going out to dinner. Going out to eat is a part of life and if you eat well during the day, it will allow you a little room when ordering off the menu.

- Know what to do at parties. All those delicious dishes at parties can pack on the pounds faster than you may think so make a point of holding a clutch purse in one hand and a glass of wine in the other–that way you do not have any hands free to nibble.

- Always take food with you when you travel–Do not go anywhere without food. You can always find a piece of fruit, nuts, or a protein bar so when the cart starts coming down the aisle with nothing but processed foods, it makes it easier to just order water with lemon or tomato juice.

- ❖ Do not allow yourself to get hungry– before you start feeling those pangs of hunger, take some time to eat ½ of a protein bar and take your time eating it. It takes a little while for your body to register that it is full and satisfied so do not rush it!

- ❖ Exercise – no matter what, find time to exercise in your day. Wake up every morning and figure out when you can exercise by taking a Pilates class or doing Yoga or lifting weights or getting on the treadmill. MAKE EXERCISE A PRIORITY and NOT AN OPTION. Would you think of going through a day without brushing your teeth or taking a shower? Think about making the time to exercise and find something you enjoy doing and look forward to it, even if it's only 20 minutes of Yoga, for example.

- ❖ Consistency is the key – do whatever it takes to stick with your plan. There are always going to be distractions or issues that arise so always have a Plan B.

- ❖ Treat yourself– if you are going to CHEAT, indulge in foods that are totally worth it. If you really want dessert,

Get in shape Small steps for big results

the low-fat version doesn't always fit the bill or satisfy the craving. Instead have a small portion of the 'real' thing. You will find that you appreciate it more when you have it in moderation.

CONCLUSION

I hope this book was able to help you understand the different ways by which you could cut down on your total body fat.

In the modern world we live in, no one has any excuse to not be in decent shape. Sure, we don't have to protect our land and hunt for our food anymore, but that doesn't mean we should look like complete and utter slobs of humans. Every single person should strive to maintain a decent level of physical fitness.

After following all the techniques discussed in this book, I guarantee you will look and feel much better. You may have to buy new clothes. You may get compliments. You may find that you love working out. One thing you will find is that you will begin to feel better and have more energy and that is the most important thing–feeling good!

Ensure that you are actually implementing the different points which you have learned in this book. We would ask you to maintain a diary which will record the whole journey. The process of losing weight is not the easiest. However, if you have done justice to the book and you actually did as I instructed, I'm confident that you must look a lot slimmer and fitter than before. Fitness has a lot of perks and you need to do all you can for the sake of shedding the pounds. With this book as a guide and the right tips with you, you should face no difficulty whatsoever in reaching your goals.

At this point you should be ready to take action and have your plan in place. Make sure you have your motivation list of benefits stuck to the fridge in big bright letters, a new shopping list of healthy goods and an organized routine of exercise which you can add to and change around as you go along. It's helpful if you knock off any smaller goals as you go along your weight loss journey to reach the ultimate goal of a happy and healthy life.

Remember to never give up and keep trying even if it seems hopeless. You will get the hang of it. Positivity and persistence is the key and it will unlock many things for you over time.

Work consistently at your program and you will see some amazing results for your efforts. You will get substantially stronger; you will shape and build your muscle and you will lose fat. After three months you'll be in a position to take your training to the next level.

Good luck in your fitness journey!

The end

Thanks for taking the time to read my book. I hope it helped you out in some type of way. If you are not already please go now and follow me here on FB here

https://www.facebook.com/RichardRobertson40/ or here https://www.instagram.com/stayingfitafter40club on Instagram.

By following me you will receive updates on all of my upcoming books, giveaways, also you will be the first to get free copies of all of my books.

Never miss another update

You can also follow me here on my Author's Page on Amazon.

Just Because

Just because you took the time to read my book here are two of my Books **FREE**. Sign up and get your books.

Forever Young: Why We Age And Proven Anti-Aging Methods

&

Staying fit after 40